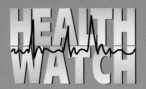

# HEALTH WATCH

# Arthritis

## *Revised Edition*

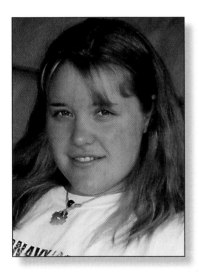

### Susan Dudley Gold

*Expert Review by Brian J. Keroack, M.D., F.A.C.R.*

**Enslow Publishers, Inc.**

40 Industrial Road          PO Box 38
Box 398                     Aldershot
Berkeley Heights, NJ 07922  Hants GU12 6BP
USA                         UK

http://www.enslow.com

*Dedicated to those who have helped me deal with rheumatoid arthritis: the members of the Pain Support Group in Saco, Maine; my son, Samuel Morrison; and my husband, John Gold; with thanks for their support and love; and to Brian J. Keroack, M.D., for his expertise and caring.*

**Acknowledgments**
With thanks to:
Brian J. Keroack, M.D., F.A.C.R., Assistant Clinical Professor of Medicine, University of Vermont; Rheumatology Associates, Portland, Maine, for his advice and review of this book.
Amanda Trask-Murphy, Laura Murphy, and Rose Spulick for their willingness to share their stories.
Donald P. Endrizzi, M.D., and Al Hardman, P.A. Orthopaedic Surgery Center, Portland, Maine, for providing information for this book.
The Arthritis Foundation for supplying photographs for this book and for offering aid and support to those with arthritis.

**Library of Congress Cataloging-in-Publication Data**
Gold, Susan Dudley.
  Arthritis / Susan Dudley Gold.—Rev. ed.
    p. cm. —— (Health watch)
Includes bibliographical references and index.
  ISBN 0-7660-1659-5 (hbk.)
    1. Arthritis—Juvenile literature. [1. Arthritis. 2. Diseases.] I. Title. II. Health watch (Berkeley Heights, N.J.)
    RC933.G58 2001
    616.7'22—dc21

                            00-010514

10 9 8 7 6 5 4 3 2 1

**To Our Readers:**
All Internet addresses in this book were active and appropriate when we went to press. Any comments or suggestions can be sent by e-mail to Comments@enslow.com or to the address on the back cover.

**Photo Credits:**
© Susan Dudley Gold: pp. 1, 4, 8, 10, 25, 41; courtesy, The Arthritis Foundation: p. 7 (*top and bottom*), p. 14 (*top and bottom*), p. 37 (Photo by John F. Smith); © PhotoDisc: p. 26; courtesy, Amanda Trask-Murphy: p. 33.
**Illustrations:**
© Susan Dudley Gold: p. 13, p. 21 (*top and bottom*); courtesy North American Precis Syndicate, Inc.: p. 34.
**Cover**
Large photo, © Susan Dudley Gold; top inset, courtesy North American Precis Syndicate, Inc.; bottom inset, © PhotoDisc.

# Contents

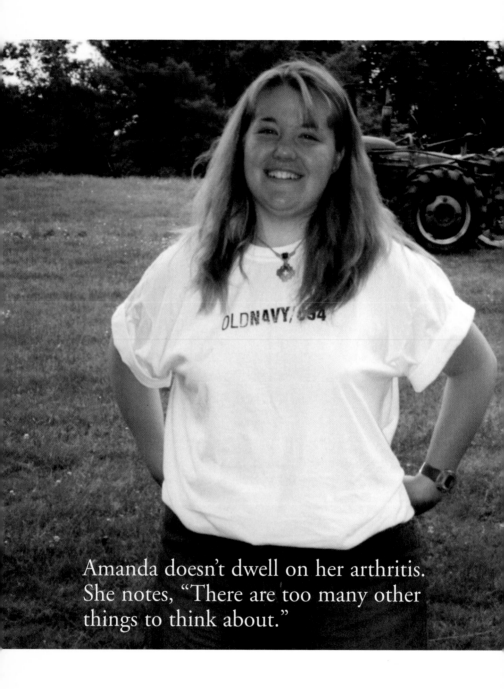

Amanda doesn't dwell on her arthritis. She notes, "There are too many other things to think about."

# Chapter 1

# Amanda's Story

Amanda Trask-Murphy was having a great time at camp. This was her third year there, and she was playing one of her favorite games, kickball. It was a hot Sunday. Most of the campers wore T-shirts and shorts. Their skin glistened with sweat as they ran to kick the ball.

But Amanda, eleven years old and looking forward to entering the fifth grade in the fall, felt cold. "I put on a sweatshirt and sweatpants, and I still felt cold," she recalls. She began to feel ill, as if she had the flu.

Finally, shivering and sick, she went to see the camp nurse. The nurse took Amanda's temperature and found she had a fever. Amanda stayed in the infirmary for the next two days. During that time, she got a rash all over her body. A local doctor gave her Tylenol and other medicine to reduce her fever. Still, Amanda's fever continued. The doctor thought she had a virus.

By Tuesday, Amanda was still feeling sick. The camp directors called her mother, who took her to the nearest doctor. "Amanda was really not well," says her mother, Laura Murphy. "She was flushed and shaking. We were sitting in the waiting room, and she said, 'W-w-when c-c-can I c-c-come in?' She couldn't even talk."

Realizing that Amanda needed special medical care, the doctor sent her to the hospital. There the doctors and nurses tested her blood, gave her antibiotic medicine to fight germs that might be in her body, and gave her fluids through a needle in her arm. Amanda stayed in the hospital for four days. Her fever went up to 104 degrees, then went down, then went up again, then went down.

After four days, doctors decided to let Amanda go home. They gave her mother medicine to help reduce Amanda's fever and make her feel better. But now Amanda had another problem: Her feet had swollen so much that her mother had trouble getting Amanda's feet into her shoes. When Amanda tried to get off the bed, the joints in her knees and feet hurt.

"It hurt her to stand on the floor," says her mother. "It hurt her to have the blankets touch her. I put my hands under her arms and helped her off the bed. It was very painful for her."

The doctors did not know what caused the swelling in Amanda's feet. The day after Amanda came home from the hospital, her fever rose again to 104 degrees. Her mother took her to the family **pediatrician**, a children's doctor. The pediatrician examined Amanda, listened to her symptoms, and said he thought she might have a form of **arthritis**.

The doctor sent Amanda to a large hospital about one hundred miles from her home. He hoped the doctors there could find out exactly what was wrong with Amanda. She stayed there for two weeks. "I could walk, but it was hard," Amanda says of that time. "My knees hurt. I couldn't run, and I couldn't write or draw."

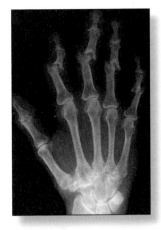

While she was in the hospital, doctors put her through many tests, including checking her blood, examining her bones and joints, and testing her urine. One day Amanda had to lie on a stretcher for a full body **X-ray**. X-ray machines use radiation to take pictures of the bones inside the body. Doctors look at the X-rays to see if a bone is broken or damaged.

In the hospital, Amanda was also examined by a **rheumatologist**, a doctor who specializes in arthritis. When the doctor saw her rash, fever, inflamed joints, and abnormal tests, he believed she had Still's disease, a form of **juvenile rheumatoid arthritis (JRA)** that affects many joints. Children with Still's disease suffer from painful swelling of the joints, skin rashes, and fever. Still's disease can cause permanent damage to the joints. It is not contagious, and

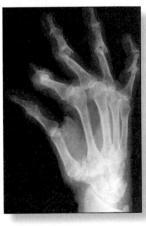

*These X-rays show bony knobs in the hands of a person with arthritis.*

Amanda did not catch it at camp. The disease was named after Dr. G.F. Still, who wrote about it in 1897.

After leaving the hospital, Amanda went to see the

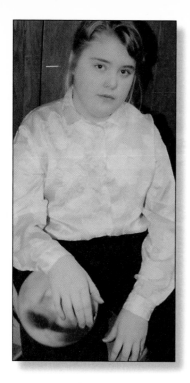

*Amanda Trask-Murphy, age thirteen, uses a ball to exercise her wrist.*

rheumatologist who had examined her. After doing more tests, he gave her several kinds of pills to take to treat the disease. He also gave her exercises to do to strengthen and stretch her muscles. Twice a week, Amanda exercises in a pool.

During the winter after the doctors found out that she had Still's disease, Amanda fell down eight times. Her joints swelled and hurt, making it hard for her to walk normally. The pain was worst in the morning. Getting out of bed was difficult. For a while, Amanda's neck was so painful that it hurt to lie in bed. Her mother remembers times when Amanda couldn't get her shoes on because her feet had swelled so much. Another time, her upper arm was so swollen that she had trouble removing her blouse.

Amanda worked on a computer at school, but ten or twenty minutes after she finished, her wrists would begin to ache. At night she wore a rubber splint on each wrist to help ease the pain. At school, she used a rubber pencil grip to help her write more easily. This soft piece of rubber wraps around the pencil and makes it easier to hold.

Amanda didn't let the disease stop her from being active. In the fall she learned how to play the saxophone and played in the school band. Since Amanda loved to read, she spent many afternoons reading mysteries at the library. Amanda also acted in plays and participated in the French club at school. Her classes included science, social studies, math, reading, writing, English, and gym.

Amanda developed a healthy attitude about her disease and learned everything she could about it. She found out that anybody of any age can have arthritis. And she didn't keep her disease a secret. Her brothers and sisters, her friends, and her classmates all knew she had the disease. When other students asked why she used a pencil grip in the classroom, "I just told them why," Amanda said.

As she entered middle school, the effects of the disease seemed to lessen. "This winter was her best," her mother said when Amanda was thirteen. After a year and a half of being on **prednisone**, one of the pills the doctor gave her to treat arthritis, Amanda was able to stop taking it.

Amanda had her blood tested every month. The tests showed how her body was reacting to the disease and to the medicine she took. Once every two months, Amanda saw her rheumatologist. He checked on the progress of the disease, asked her how she was feeling, and questioned her about pain, rashes, and any problems she had had. During her spring checkup when she was thirteen, the doctor told her that she was the best she had been since she got the disease.

Amanda turned thirteen two years after she found out she had arthritis. By then, the medicine and the exercise had helped her. "It's made me feel a lot better," said Amanda. "When I was first sick, I couldn't do a lot of things, but now I can do everything I used to do."

Amanda has made amazing progress. But she still has

difficult times. For example, she had been feeling so well that she decided to march with her band in a state parade. The marching made Amanda's symptoms worse. "The parade wasn't too long," her mother said, "but it was too long for Amanda. It was too much for her."

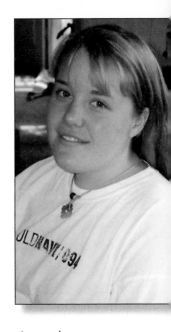

For three weeks after the parade, Amanda's right side was swollen, she had a fever, and her thighs hurt. After school, she came home exhausted and went to bed.

But her mother is encouraged by Amanda's improvement over the years. "She's been doing really well," Mrs. Murphy said. Since this book was first written, Amanda's disease has gone into **remission**. That means she no longer has any symptoms, and she

*Amanda, age eighteen. Her arthritis has been in remission for four years.*

doesn't have to take medication for arthritis. Amanda's joints still ache when she overdoes, though. After a long day of shopping, her knees and feet swelled and she developed a rash along the painful joints. The doctors don't know enough about the disease to predict how Amanda will do later. They are hoping that she will continue to do well.

"This is a lifelong thing," says Mrs. Murphy. "Amanda is not going to get all better in a year. But she doesn't want to give in. She's a very strong-willed child and that's been good for her."

# Chapter 2

# What Is Arthritis?

Almost 43 million Americans suffer from some form of arthritis. Of those, nearly three hundred thousand are children. About fifty thousand children have the most severe form of juvenile rheumatoid arthritis. According to doctors at the national Centers for Disease Control in Atlanta, Georgia, arthritis is the number one health problem for adult women in this country.

Arthritis is not contagious. Other people cannot catch it from someone who has the disease. Most forms of arthritis are chronic, which means they last a long time, usually for life. There is no cure, and scientists don't know for sure what causes arthritis. Symptoms appear and then may disappear. A few people have only one or two attacks of arthritis and then never have it again. Other people have pain for the rest of their lives.

People have suffered from arthritis for centuries. It is one of the oldest diseases known. Signs of arthritis have even been found in Egyptian mummies. The early Romans built a system of warm baths to ease arthritis pain.

Many famous people have had arthritis. Christopher Columbus; Mary, Queen of Scots; and our eighth president, James Madison, all had some form of the disease. Former First Lady Betty Ford, pro football star Dick Butkus, and movie star Elizabeth Taylor are notable figures who have arthritis.

The word *arthritis* means "inflammation of the joint." Many, but not all, forms of arthritis cause joints to swell. But all forms of arthritis involve problems with joints.

Joints can be found wherever two bones meet. They allow people to bend, move, wave, run, walk, and chew. A joint is made up of six parts:

1. **Cartilage** On the end of each bone, wherever it meets another bone, is a thin layer of tough tissue called cartilage. The cartilage is like a rubber cushion that keeps the bones from rubbing against each other.

2. **Muscle** The muscles, which are connected to the bones, are made up of tissues that bunch up, or contract. When these muscles contract, bones move.

3. **Tendon** Tendons are the tough, fibrous bands of tissue that connect the muscles to the bones.

4. **Ligament** Shorter bands of tough tissue, called ligaments, connect bones to other bones. The outer part of the joint is made up of ligaments.

5. **Synovial sac** The synovial sac is a thin tissue that lines the joint. It is filled with a fluid that works like oil in a car, lubricating the joint and making it move easily.

6. **Bursa** Near the joint is the bursa, a small sac of fluid. The fluid oils the muscles and keeps them moving smoothly.

People with arthritis have something wrong with a part

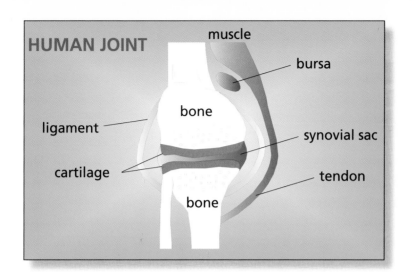

*A human joint is shown.*

of the joint. For example, people with **osteoarthritis (OA)** have problems with cartilage. In the joints of those with OA, the cartilage starts to wear away, causing their bones to rub together.

The synovial sac is affected in those with **rheumatoid arthritis (RA)**. The sac swells, which damages the rest of the joint. People with **ankylosing spondylitis (AS)** have swelling where the ligaments join to the bone.

There are one hundred twenty-seven known forms of arthritis. The disease affects infants as well as the elderly and people of all ages in between. Arthritis falls into two main groups: degenerative and inflammatory. There are also other diseases, discussed later in this book, that are closely related to arthritis.

## Degenerative Arthritis

Rose Spulick was thirty years old when she learned she had osteoarthritis. Osteoarthritis is a form of **degenerative**

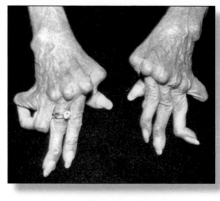

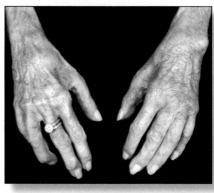

**arthritis**. Rose recalls baking cupcakes one morning for her son's kindergarten class. As she stood in her kitchen and tried to frost the cakes, she burst into tears because her lower spine hurt so much.

Degenerative arthritis is the most common type of arthritis. In most cases, there is little swelling with this kind of arthritis. It is often called the wear-and-tear disease. Heavy use of joints over a long period of time or being overweight can put pressure on the joints. Joints that have been injured in the past develop osteoarthritis more quickly than other joints. That is why some athletes get OA as they grow older.

*Surgery can help some people with the severest forms of arthritis. These photos show an extreme example of deformity caused by arthritis and the improvement after surgery.*

Almost everyone who lives to be eighty or ninety has some type of degenerative arthritis, usually OA. But younger people can also have the disease.

In many people, OA damages the cartilage in the hips or the knees. Without a cushion of cartilage, the bones rub against each other. This causes pain and can interfere with movement. In cases where the hips or knees are badly damaged, doctors may replace the joints with metal ones.

In another form of OA, people develop knobs in the finger joints. These bony knobs are called **Heberden's nodes**. The fingers may become stiff, but usually the knobs don't cause other problems. Women are much more likely than men to have Heberden's nodes.

OA can also affect the spine. People with this problem develop bony growths or spurs along their spines. The spurs can pinch the nerves running from the brain down the spine to other parts of the body. This can cause pain and make it hard for people to move well.

## Inflammatory Arthritis

Swelling and pain in the joints are the marks of **inflammatory arthritis**. In this type of arthritis, something causes the white blood cells in the joint to divide and grow. The white blood cells attack the joint, releasing chemicals that cause it to swell and feel hot. Over time, both the cartilage and the bone can be destroyed.

Rheumatoid arthritis is the most common form of inflammatory arthritis. About 2.1 million Americans have the disease, and almost three-quarters of them are women.

The disease causes pain, stiffness, and swelling in the joints. A person with RA feels tired, stiff, and sore, and often has trouble walking or moving around. He or she may have **anemia**, a condition in which the number of red blood cells is lower than normal. Anemia makes a person weak and tired. RA can also affect a person's muscles, lungs, heart, blood vessels, skin, eyes, and nerves.

RA causes swelling of the synovial sac lining the joint. This swelling causes pain and redness. Eventually, the swelling can damage the whole joint. If it is not treated, RA can cause people's fingers to curl. People with severe RA may need to use a wheelchair. RA in its most severe form does more damage to the joints than any other type of arthritis.

Juvenile rheumatoid arthritis is a form of inflammatory arthritis that strikes children. Like Amanda Trask-Murphy, young children and teenagers with this kind of arthritis suffer from swollen joints, pain, and stiffness. As with RA in adults, JRA usually affects joints on both sides of the body.

There are three types of JRA: pauciarticular, polyarticular, and systemic. In **pauciarticular JRA**, only one or two joints, usually in the legs, are affected. It most often occurs in girls under the age of ten.

**Polyarticular JRA** affects five or more joints. A child with this form of the disease may have a fever and have lumps under the skin. This type of JRA causes the most damage to the joints if it is not treated. Girls are more likely to get this type of JRA.

About 30 percent of children with juvenile rheumatoid arthritis have **systemic JRA**, which affects the whole system. It is also called Still's disease, the type of JRA affecting Amanda. Both boys and girls get Still's disease. Like Amanda, those with the disease have a high fever at first. Every joint in their bodies swells and hurts. Children with the disease may have a rash.

Still's disease may also affect the heart, the liver, the spleen, and the kidneys. These problems can be treated and may go away after a few months.

Ankylosing spondylitis is another form of inflammatory arthritis. In cases of AS, swelling occurs where the tendons and ligaments attach to the bone. The swelling is so severe in some cases that it destroys the cartilage. If this happens, the bones in the spine may fuse together. The disease usually strikes people between the ages of twenty and forty years. It is most common in young men. Ankylosing spondylitis is a form of **seronegative spondyloarthropathy**, a type of disease that causes inflammation throughout the body, especially in the spine and joints. The first sign of ankylosing spondylitis is pain in the lower back. People who have severe AS cannot bend their backs.

**Reactive arthritis**, also a form of seronegative spondyloarthropathy, was first described by two French physicians during World War I. Many soldiers became sick with an infection called dysentery. Then their joints began to hurt. They had eye problems, painful heels, and pain while urinating. Sufferers also developed a rash.

Reactive arthritis is the most common form of arthritis in young men. Women and older people can get the disease, too. Scientists think reactive arthritis is caused by infection. The infection is usually linked to diarrhea, food poisoning, salmonella (germs found in food), or venereal diseases (diseases caused by sexual contact).

**Lyme disease** is an illness caused by a tick bite. A tick is a tiny animal related to the spider. Some ticks are the size of the period at the end of this sentence. The tick infects the body with germs called bacteria. The infection can lead to arthritis, causing the joints to swell and ache. It can also affect the brain and the heart. A person with Lyme disease often feels as if he or she has the flu. Lyme disease can be treated with antibiotics. If it is not treated quickly, though, the flare-ups may continue.

# Related Diseases

**Lupus (systemic lupus erythematosus)** is an inflammatory disease that can be extremely painful. Like RA, it causes swollen joints and can affect muscles, skin, nerves, lungs, and other organs. Unlike RA, lupus does not destroy the bone in the joint.

People with lupus often get tired, feel weak, and lose weight. They may have a rash on the face, neck, or arms. Muscle aches, sores in the nose or mouth, loss of hair, and swollen glands are also common. Some people have seizures and suffer from heart, liver, and kidney problems related to lupus. Symptoms may come and go. Sometimes a person with lupus feels fine. In severe cases, he or she may have to stay in the hospital for treatment.

Approximately 90 percent of lupus cases involve women between eighteen and forty-five years old. Men, young children, and older adults can also get the disease. About five hundred thousand Americans have been diagnosed with lupus. It is most common among African-Americans, Native Americans, Chinese, Hispanics, and Filipinos.

**Fibromyalgia** affects the soft tissue around the joints. It is estimated that about 20 percent of patients treated by arthritis doctors have this disease. It strikes mostly women between twenty and sixty, although men can also have the disease. People with fibromyalgia feel pain throughout the body. Pressing certain points on the body triggers pain. The disease keeps people from sleeping well and causes them to feel weak and tired. Muscles are stiff, especially in the morning. Fibromyalgia does not cause lasting damage to the joints.

# Chapter 3

# Causes and Diagnosis

N
o one knows for sure what causes arthritis. People used to think that degenerative arthritis was caused by the movements of bones over a lifetime. But doctors now know that moderate exercise helps keep joints healthy.

When a joint is injured, the injury may lead to osteoarthritis. An injury can damage the cartilage. Or an injury can make movement of the joint painful. If the joint does not get much use, it will not receive the oxygen and nutrients it needs to stay healthy. Over time, the cartilage becomes thin and wears away.

In younger people, osteoarthritis appears to be linked to a person's **genes**. Genes are tiny units within each cell that determine a person's features. People inherit genes from both their mothers and their fathers. Genes determine whether a person's eyes are blue or brown and whether his or her hair is straight or curly. Genes can also pass along a tendency to get certain diseases. Researchers have found that people like Rose Spulick often have a defect or mistake in the genes governing their cartilage that makes it wear out sooner.

Scientists have other ideas about what causes inflammatory diseases like rheumatoid arthritis. Some think a virus or some type of germ may trigger the disease.

The purpose of the **immune system** is to protect the body from germs and disease. When a germ invades the body, the immune system sends out an alarm. Alerted to the invader (also called an **antigen**), white blood cells begin to divide and grow. Soon an army of **antibodies**, a type of protein made by the white blood cells, attacks the invader. This causes inflammation, which is why a person's finger swells when it gets infected. The antibodies rush to the area to protect the body from the germs causing the infection.

Other white blood cells called **macrophages** arrive on the scene and eat the invader. Then, once the invader is destroyed, a special type of white blood cell called a **suppressor cell** signals the body to stop the attack.

Sometimes, though, the body gets confused. Its white blood cells may begin the attack on a germ as usual. But after the germ is gone, the cells may attack the body itself. In other cases, the cells may confuse a part of the body with a germ. If this happens, the white blood cells may launch an attack on that part of the body.

In the case of rheumatoid arthritis, researchers think a virus may activate the immune system. Then, for some unknown reason, the white blood cells attack the synovial sac that lines the joints. If the attack is not stopped, the

# IMMUNE RESPONSE

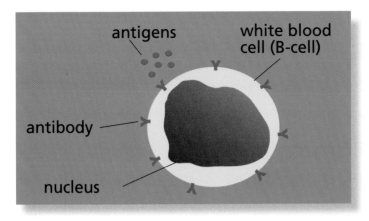

*Above, the B-cell's antibodies defend the body against the antigens that have invaded the bloodstream.*

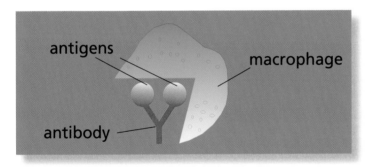

*Here, the antigens become attached to the antibodies and then are surrounded and destroyed by the macrophage.*

cartilage and bone in the joint will be seriously damaged or destroyed.

Researchers think people may be affected differently by viruses and other germs. For example, one virus may trigger RA in one person and leave another person unaffected. The difference may be due to a person's genes.

Some people with RA have a spot on a gene that most people do not have. This spot is called a **genetic marker**. The genetic marker, **HLA-DR4**, is found in about 75 percent of people with RA. Doctors think that people with

HLA-DR4 may be more likely than others to get RA if they are exposed to a certain virus.

But some people with the marker do not develop RA. Others without the marker do develop it. Why? Scientists do not know.

Stress may play a role in RA and other diseases in which the immune system doesn't work right. For example, doctors report that arthritis becomes worse in some patients who are under stress.

Amanda was doing much better until she went through a stressful time. All at once her feet began to swell again, she got a rash, and she was in pain. "It was very evident that [the flare-up] was stress-related," said Mrs. Murphy.

Scientists think the immune system may also be to blame in diseases such as lupus, ankylosing spondylitis, and reactive arthritis.

## Making a Diagnosis

With so many known types of arthritis, how does a doctor determine what type a patient has? It can be difficult, especially in the early stages, to diagnose arthritis. Like Amanda, people often have to go through many tests and see several doctors before the right diagnosis is made.

Doctors use a number of tools and tests to find the answers. First, doctors conduct a complete physical exam. They look for signs of swollen joints, hot areas, rashes, and other symptoms. It is also important to rule out other diseases.

But most of all, doctors depend on their patients to tell them what is wrong. By reporting how the disease affects them, patients can often give enough clues to lead to the right diagnosis.

One of the best ways to find out if a person has OA is to X-ray the joints that are painful. An X-ray shows the position and the condition of the bones. It can also reveal bony growths in the fingers or along the spine that can be the result of osteoarthritis.

X-rays do not show cartilage. An X-ray of a healthy joint will show two bones separated by a space. The space is where the cartilage is located. A joint damaged by OA will show only a narrow space or a thin line between the two bones. That means only a thin layer of cartilage—sometimes no cartilage—separates the bones.

Inflammatory arthritis, such as rheumatoid arthritis, is harder to identify. In many cases, little damage to the cartilage or bone occurs until late in the disease. Therefore, X-rays are not helpful in making an early diagnosis.

Tests can help. About 80 percent of people with RA have what is called the **rheumatoid factor** in their blood. The rheumatoid factor is a type of antibody. Some doctors think the body makes the antibody to help fight RA. Others believe that the antibody may play some role in causing RA. Oddly, some people who do not have RA do have the rheumatoid factor. And some people who have RA do not have the factor or may have it only later in the course of the disease.

Another blood test used to diagnose arthritis measures how fast red blood cells settle to the bottom of a tube. This is called the **sed rate**. If the blood cells settle too quickly, that means the person probably has inflammation that might be caused by arthritis. Though the test won't reveal the type of arthritis, it will show how active the disease is. Another test analyzes the fluid in the joint. A high number of white blood cells shows that the joint is inflamed. A test for C-reactive protein, a protein that increases when rheumatoid arthritis is active, is also useful in diagnosing and treating the disease.

Doctors also test patients' blood to see whether they have anemia. This is a sign of RA and some other forms of inflammatory arthritis.

A number of tests have been developed to test for lupus. One is the anti-nuclear antibody (ANA) test. People with lupus have a high concentration of ANA. But no test by itself is proof of the disease. People who do not have lupus sometimes have a high ANA reading. Other types of blood tests are also helpful in diagnosing lupus. But some people with lupus may have normal tests, while people who do not have the disease may test positive. Some people may test positive one time and negative another time.

In making a diagnosis, doctors also look for certain symptoms such as aching joints, swelling, stiffness that is worse in the morning, joints that feel hot to the touch, and unexplained weight loss, fever, or weakness. But many of the symptoms can be caused by other diseases. It can take months, sometimes years, before doctors know for sure what disease the patient has.

In RA and some other forms of arthritis, people have genetic markers that show up in tests. Ankylosing spondylitis and reactive arthritis are linked to a genetic marker, **HLA-B27**. A person with other symptoms of either of these diseases may be tested for HLA-B27 to help confirm the diagnosis.

# Chapter 4

# Care and Treatment

There is no cure for arthritis. But there are many treatments that can help people with arthritis feel better. The treatment depends on the kind of arthritis and the person's health needs.

## Exercise

Almost everyone who has arthritis benefits from exercise. Even joints that are painful need to be exercised. If they are kept still too long, the muscles become weak and the cartilage thins. But the exercise must be gentle enough not to cause more damage. Swimming is especially good

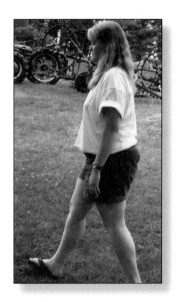

*Amanda, age eighteen, enjoys swimming and going for walks to keep in shape.*

for people with arthritis because it doesn't put weight on the joints. Walking and working with exercise machines are also helpful. Amanda walks and swims to keep in shape.

## Special Devices

There are many devices to help people with arthritis. Canes, crutches, and walkers help people move more easily and safely. Grip bars make it easier to walk up stairs or get into and out of the bathtub.

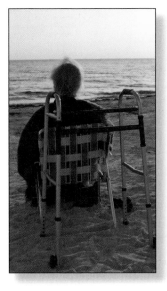

Special tools for the kitchen help people with arthritis do things for themselves. Those who have trouble turning their wrists benefit from special door handles and knobs on sinks and cupboards. Amanda used a pencil grip to make writing less painful. In school she typed on an electric typewriter and later on a computer.

*Walkers and other devices help people with arthritis live more normal lives.*

## Diet and Lifestyle

There is no special diet that has been proven to cure arthritis. But a healthy diet that is low in fat can help people to stay trim and feel well. Excess weight can put pressure on joints and make them hurt even more.

Rest is important for people with arthritis. The disease often leaves those who have it feeling tired. Because stress can cause flare-ups, people with arthritis need to learn how to relax. People can also learn how to use their joints to avoid hurting them.

## Medicine

For Amanda, prednisone was "a miracle drug," her mother said. Before she took it, Amanda had to have help from her mother to dress, walk, and even comb her hair. Once the medicine began to work, Amanda was able to move more easily and take care of herself. "The first thing I noticed," recalled her mother, "was that she began to comb her hair and put rollers in it. When she got up in the morning, she could move faster."

There are four basic types of medicine for arthritis: pain-relievers; drugs that reduce swelling, called **non-steroidal anti-inflammatory drugs (NSAIDs)**; artificial hormones called **corticosteroids**; and **disease-modifying anti-rheumatic drugs (DMARDs)**.

Tylenol or other painkillers may be all that people with a mild case of arthritis need. For others, though, stronger medicine may be required. NSAIDs help relieve the pain and also reduce swelling. Aspirin is the best-known NSAID. It is used in high doses (twelve to twenty-four pills a day) to reduce swelling in people with inflammatory arthritis, like RA. Ibuprofen (Advil, Motrin) and naproxen (Naprosyn, Aleve) are some other NSAIDs.

All the arthritis medicines have side effects. Aspirin and other NSAIDs can cause stomach ulcers, nausea, and ringing in the ears. Doctors often advise patients to drink milk or eat food when the pills are taken. Drinking or eating coats the stomach and helps ease digestive problems.

Corticosteroids were first introduced in the 1950s as an arthritis treatment. Prednisone is the most widely used steroid for arthritis. It is an artificial hormone that is like some produced by the body. Prednisone helps reduce inflammation and swelling. Corticosteroids are not like the steroids taken by some athletes, which are more like natural male hormones.

When a person suffering from a bad case of inflammatory arthritis takes prednisone, the swelling and pain can stop almost at once. Steroids can be taken in pill form or in injections. A shot of steroid into a swollen joint may ease the pain for a day or for several months.

But steroids can also cause problems when taken for a long time. Amanda gained fifty pounds while taking prednisone. Steroids can cause bones to thin, blood pressure to rise, depression, and vision problems. For these reasons, doctors try to limit the amount of steroids patients use.

People with RA, lupus, and other diseases of the immune system may need another form of medicine, DMARDs. While other types of medicine can offer relief, they cannot stop the disease from destroying the joints. DMARDs can slow and sometimes stop joint damage altogether. Doctors are not sure exactly how the medicines work. But they know DMARDs change the disease in some way. Most of DMARDs take three months or more to work. In some patients the effects of the disease can disappear while the patient is taking the medicine.

There are several types of DMARDs. One type is made up of chemicals that contain gold. Sometimes called gold salts, such medicines have been used to control RA since the 1920s. They come in a liquid or pill form that can be taken by mouth. Gold salts can also be injected. Some people use these medicines for years.

Plaquenil is a DMARD that was first used to treat malaria, a tropical disease. It is used in RA and lupus patients to reduce swelling and slow the disease.

**Methotrexate** is the DMARD used most often by RA patients. It is also used to treat lupus, juvenile rheumatoid arthritis, and other types of arthritis. Methotrexate is also used in higher doses as an anti-cancer drug. The medicine slows and sometimes stops the immune cells from attacking the synovial sac. But it can also reduce the body's ability to fight off germs.

As with other medicines, DMARDs have side effects. They can cause nausea, blisters, and rashes. Plaquenil can also lead to vision problems. More serous problems are rare. They include blindness and liver and kidney damage. Doctors test patients' blood every few weeks and perform other examinations to make sure no serious damage is being caused by the DMARDs.

## New Treatments

Several new medications—and some supplements—have given people with arthritis hope in their fight against the disease. Researchers have developed new medicines for arthritis patients that are less likely to cause ulcers and stomach upsets than NSAIDs. These drugs, called **COX-2 inhibitors,** reduce inflammation and ease pain. Two—celecoxib (Celebrex) and rofecoxib (Vioxx)—received approval from the Federal Drug Administration in 1999. A third—meloxicam (Mobic)—was under review in 2000.

Some osteoarthritis patients have been helped by glucosamine sulfate and chondroitin, substances that occur naturally in the body and that are involved in repairing and protecting cartilage. Glucosamine supplements are made from the shells of shellfish. An extract from the windpipes of cattle is used to make chondroitin supplements. Several studies have shown that the supplements help ease swelling and pain caused by osteoarthritis. Now a $6.6 million study by the National Institutes of Health will investigate whether the supplements can also stop damage to cartilage in OA patients.

Even more strides have been made in the fight against rheumatoid arthritis. Leflunomide (Arava), a DMARD approved in the late 1990s, blocks certain white blood cells that cause inflammation in RA patients. Taken as a pill, the new medication has helped people who found no relief from methotrexate or who couldn't take the older drug because of its side effects.

Two of the newest medicines—etanercept (Enbrel) and infliximab (Remicade)—have also reduced swelling, eased pain, and stopped joint damage in some people with arthritis. Both are **biologic agents**—proteins that target chemicals in the body. These medicines absorb a chemical that increases inflammation called **tumor necrosis factor (TNF)**. Unlike older medicines such as methotrexate that suppress the entire immune system, these new drugs act only on the offending chemicals.

Etanercept was first offered to adult patients in the United States in 1999. The following year doctors began using it on young patients. Patients inject etanercept under the skin with a small needle twice a week. The results have been dramatic in some people with severe rheumatoid arthritis. Etanercept enabled one teenage girl who had been confined to a wheelchair and in almost constant pain to join the school swim team. Before taking the medicine, almost every joint in her body was swollen.

The medicine works by blocking proteins called cytokines. Cytokines are proteins used by cells to communicate with one another. Some increase inflammation, while others decrease inflammation. Etanercept blocks TNF, a cytokine that increases inflammation. This can also be a drawback, however. Doctors worry that patients on etanercept may develop infections because the drug may make the body less able to fight off germs. Because of this, only people with severe forms of the disease who have not been helped by other medicines are given etanercept.

Infliximab, which works much as etanercept does, also blocks TNF. Approved for RA in late 1999, it is combined with methotrexate and given intravenously once a month or every other month. Both infliximab and etanercept are expensive. Etanercept costs about $1,190 for a month's supply. Infliximab's price tag is slightly more than $1,200 for an eight-week dose plus the cost of IV treatment.

A few people with moderate to severe rheumatoid arthritis have benefited from another option, called protein A immunoadsorption therapy or Prosorba treatment. Those undergoing the therapy have blood drawn from one arm. A special machine separates the liquid, or plasma, from the blood cells. The plasma is then processed to remove the antibodies. After the processing, the plasma and the blood cells are mixed together again and injected into a vein in the patient's other arm. This treatment is still experimental and has not proven to be effective for many people. The therapy can cost as much as $18,000 for the full twelve-week course.

## Alternative Methods

Not everyone with arthritis is helped by medicine. Some people may even get sick from taking medicines. Others can't find one that works for them. Even those who get relief from medicines may also benefit from other methods of treatment. By combining certain methods, some people can reduce the amount of medicine they take.

**Acupuncture** is an ancient Eastern form of treatment that was developed in Asia, especially China. In this treatment, tiny needles are inserted into the body at certain points. People who practice acupuncture believe the needles help energy flow more easily through the body. Scientists in the United States and other western countries agree that acupuncture helps some people with painful joints and back problems. But the scientists don't understand how acupuncture works.

**Massage therapy** is another ancient form of treatment. Trained therapists rub the muscles in the body. This can help people relax and feel better.

For some people, ice packs make swollen joints feel better. Others find that a heating pad or a soak in warm water helps to ease their pain. In another treatment, people dip their hands or feet in hot wax. Once they are coated, the hands or feet are wrapped with a towel until the wax cools.

A device called a **TENS unit** works for some people. The unit gives off a small electrical current. This passes through a person's nerves and prevents pain signals from reaching the brain.

Because tense muscles can make pain worse, relaxing is helpful for people with arthritis. **Biofeedback** teaches people how to relax. Using a machine, people learn to control their blood pressure and body temperature and to relax tense muscles. Other ways to relax include meditating, deep breathing, and self-hypnosis.

## Support From Others

A positive attitude can make anyone feel better. Sometimes it helps people to talk with others who have the same kind of problem. In support groups, people share ways of living with arthritis. They learn about other methods to ease pain. And they learn that they are not alone.

Amanda attended a summer camp in Vermont for children with arthritis for several summers. There she met other children and teens who had arthritis. "That was one of the best things she did," said her mother, Laura Murphy. "She thought she was the only one who had arthritis. When she got to camp, there was a whole camp full of kids with the disease." Several of the camp counselors had arthritis, too. "They showed her what people with arthritis could do," said Mrs. Murphy.

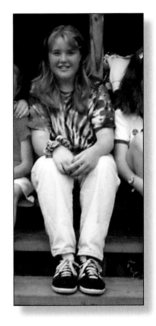

*Amanda, age fourteen, sits with friends at arthritis summer camp.*

# Chapter 5

# New Joints for an Arthritic Body

Sometimes nothing can stop arthritis from damaging a joint. When that happens, doctors can replace a natural joint with an artificial metal one. This helps ease the pain and lets patients move more easily.

Every year, more than five hundred thousand people in the United States have joints replaced. Doctors can replace joints in the shoulder, elbow, hip, knee, and finger. People have knees and hips replaced most often.

Joint replacement can bring amazing results. One woman with arthritis could hardly walk. She

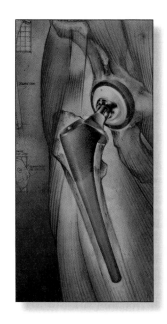

*A hip replacement is shown inside the body.*

34

had two shoulders, two hips, two knees, and one ankle replaced. After all the operations, she was able to dance.

Let's look in on a knee replacement operation. The patient is lying on the operating table. He has been given medicine so that he can't feel any pain, but he is awake. The doctor is replacing the patient's left knee. She carefully cuts the skin below and above the knee and then peels it back to see the bones.

She sees the femur (thigh bone) and the tibia (shin bone) where they join at the patient's knee. But the cartilage that covers the ends of both bones, and normally acts as a cushion whenever the patient takes a step, is seriously damaged. There are bloody holes in the cartilage where it has been eaten away. In other spots it has been worn thin. The damage has been caused by rheumatoid arthritis.

The doctor has quite a selection of tools. One might almost think her toolbox belonged to a carpenter. She uses a tool called a rongeur to clear away the tissue and cartilage left around the bone. The rongeur looks like a pair of scissors. But instead of snipping the tissue, it bites it away.

Then the doctor picks up a special electric saw. With a buzz, the saw cuts a quarter of an inch off the bottom and the sides of the femur. The doctor trims another quarter of an inch off the top of the tibia. The ends of these bones, which were round, are now flat.

Now it's time for the patient to see his new knee. The part that connects to the femur is shaped like a yo-yo. It has two identical, rounded metal parts that are made of a **titanium** alloy, a shiny, lightweight but strong metal. Titanium is also used in aircraft and in space vehicles.

The part connected to the tibia looks like a plastic dish.

It will fit on the bottom of the "yo-yo." Together the two pieces will create a knee for the patient.

The replacement knees are made in a factory. Most people can use the same size. A few people, who have odd-shaped knees, have to have special replacements custom-made for them.

The surgeon puts cement on the flat end of the femur. The cement is like the glue a dentist uses to attach fillings to teeth. Once the cement is applied, the doctor uses a short hammer to pound the yo-yo onto the femur.

Then she hammers a metal holder with a peg into the tibia. She covers the metal holder with cement, then places the plastic dish on the holder.

Once the cement is dry, the doctor tests the new knee. She does this by putting the skin back in place, bending the knee, and then straightening it. If the knee doesn't work just right, she trims some fat or tissue from around it so that the bones move smoothly. Then she sews up the skin. The operation takes about one and one-half hours.

Joint replacements are among the most common operations performed. In 90 percent of the cases, they ease pain and help patients move more easily. One woman with RA said her shoulder felt better than it had for years—even though she had undergone joint surgery just the day before.

One drawback of this kind of surgery is that the new joint usually comes unglued after about fifteen years. Researchers are trying to find other ways to attach the joint to the bone. In younger patients, doctors sometimes use a joint with a coating filled with tiny holes. The bone can grow into the holes and hold the joint in place.

In other patients, the plastic dish wears out. Researchers are testing the use of ceramics in artificial joints instead of metal. They hope that ceramic ball joints will cause less wear and tear on the plastic dish that serves as a socket.

Soon after the surgery is finished, the patient must begin an exercise program. This helps the muscles that move the bones around the joint get back in shape. Some patients can start exercising a day or two after surgery.

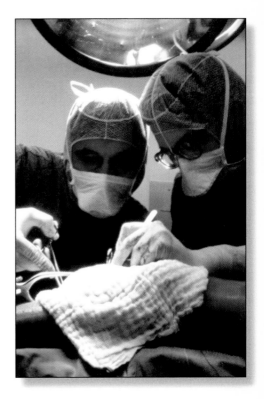

*Surgeons replace an arthritic knee with a metal one.*

Even though joint replacements don't last forever, they can help people with arthritis live normal lives for many years. The woman with seven metal joints would certainly testify to that!

# Chapter 6

# Research: Hope for Tomorrow

Exciting progress has been made in the last few years in the fight against arthritis. Osteoarthritis patients have new medicines that ease pain and have fewer side effects. Researchers have discovered new medicines and treatments that slow rheumatoid arthritis. The newest medicines target specific parts of the immune system to prevent swelling and damage to joints.

People with arthritis can get new joints to replace diseased ones. New devices have been created to help those with arthritis live more normal lives. People have learned to use ancient remedies like massage and acupuncture to help ease the pain.

Some researchers have used bone marrow transplants in children with severe rheumatoid arthritis. Stem cells from the transplants have grown new immune systems in the children in the test. So far, none of the children have had any signs of arthritis. Scientists don't know exactly why this procedure works, but they continue their studies in the hope that someday such techniques may prevent or cure arthritis.

Research on glucosamine and chondroitin show that these supplements may slow down or stop cartilage damage caused by osteoarthritis. Scientists are also testing ways to regrow cartilage that has been damaged. European tests have shown that healthy cartilage may be grown in damaged joints in athletes. In Connecticut, a company is using magnetic rays to regrow cartilage damaged by osteoarthritis. Scientists continue to test these methods.

Good scientists always test their findings over and over to make sure the results are true. When they work with a new drug, they test it first on animals. If the tests work out well, scientists then try the drug on humans.

The drug to be tested is given to one group of patients. An inactive pill, or **placebo**, is given to another group. The placebo looks like the real thing, but it does not contain the medicine in the test drug. For example, some placebos contain only sugar water.

In a **double-blind test**, neither the patients nor their doctors know whether the drug or a placebo is being used. Some people get better whenever they take any medicine, even a placebo. This happens because the people *believe* they will get better, and their minds help them to feel better, if only for a while. This is called the **placebo effect**. If the group taking the real drug does better than the group taking the placebo, there is evidence that the drug may work. Doctors do many tests on a large number of people to see whether the drug works and if it has harmful side effects.

# Quack Cures

Quack cures for arthritis have been around as long as people have suffered from the disease. A device known as a Cosmos bag—full of radioactive ore—was said to ease the pain from arthritis when placed on sore joints. It was sold in the early 1900s. Another device shaped like a nail and marketed in the time of George Washington claimed to relieve arthritis when dragged across bare skin.

In too many cases, people try to sell expensive, fake cures to those who have arthritis. There is no cure for arthritis yet, but people who are in pain want to believe that a cure has been found. Often they will try anything to get relief.

Some of these "treatments," like wearing a copper bracelet, are harmless as well as useless. Others, however, can be costly, useless, and dangerous. Snake venom and bee venom are claimed to help people with arthritis. But both can cause serious allergic reactions.

Some people decide to use unproven remedies instead of the medicines given to them by their doctor. This can cause their disease to become active again. In some cases, it can lead to serious problems. One doctor tells of a lupus patient who lost the use of her kidneys after she stopped the treatment her doctor had prescribed.

Arthritis symptoms can come and go by themselves. Sometimes people's symptoms will disappear at the same time they are taking an unproven remedy. Then they think the remedy—for example, herbs or vitamins or a strange diet—made them better. The Arthritis Foundation tells people to check carefully the research done on arthritis treatments. Treatments must be tested on many people to tell for sure if they work.

A cure for arthritis—when it is found—most certainly will not be announced in a television commercial. The news will appear under giant headlines on the front page of the newspaper.

Until then, people with arthritis must live their lives as best they can, helped by new joints, effective medicines, special devices, and positive attitudes.

Since this book was first written, Amanda Trask-Murphy has graduated with honors from high school and will attend Johnson and Wales University in Providence, Rhode Island. She will study culinary arts and hopes to be a pastry chef someday. Amanda doesn't dwell on her arthritis. She notes, "There are too many other things to think about."

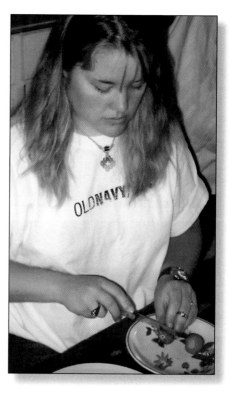

*Amanda prepares strawberries for dessert. She will attend college, where she plans to study culinary arts.*

# Further Reading

Adams, Pam. *Disabled People*. Auburn, Maine: Child's Play, 1990.

Aldape, Virginia Tortorica, et al. *Nicole's Story: A Book About a Girl With Juvenile Rheumatoid Arthritis*. Minneapolis: Lerner Publications, 1996.

Arthritis Foundation. *Decision Making for Teenagers With Arthritis*. Atlanta, Ga.: Arthritis Foundation, 1999.

Brewer, Earl J. Jr., M.D., and Kathy Cochran Angel. *The Arthritis Sourcebook: Everything You Need to Know*. Los Angeles: Lowell House, 1994.

Brewer, Earl J. Jr., M.D., Edward H. Giannini, et al. *Juvenile Rheumatoid Arthritis*. Los Angeles: Lowell House, 1993.

Kriegsman, Kay H., et al. *Taking Charge: Teenagers Talk About Life & Physical Disabilities*. Bethesda, Md.: Woodbine House, 1992.

Moyer, Ellen. *Arthritis: Questions You Have—Answers You Need*. Allentown, Penn.: Peoples Medical Society, 1993.

Peacock, Judith. *Juvenile Arthritis*. Santa Rosa, Calif.: Lifematters, 2000.

Shenkman, John. *Living With Arthritis (Living With Series)*. New York: Franklin Watts, 1990.

White, Peter. *Disabled People*. New York: Franklin Watts, 1990.

Willett, Edward. *Arthritis*. Berkeley Heights, N.J.: Enslow Publishers, 2000.

# For More Information

The following is a list of resources that deal with arthritis.

## Organizations

**Arthritis Foundation**
1330 West Peachtree St., Atlanta, GA 30309, (404) 872-7100; <http://www.arthritis.org>. (Look in the telephone book for your local chapter.)

**Spondylitis Association**
14827 Ventura Blvd. # 222, Sherman Oaks, CA 91403; <http://www.spondylitis.org>.

**Lupus Foundation of America**
1300 Piccard Drive, Suite 200, Rockville, MD 20850; (800) 558-0121; <http://www.lupus.org>.

## Internet Resources

**<http://www.aaos.org>**
American Academy of Orthopaedic Surgeons.

**<http://www.aphanet.org>**
American Pharmaceutical Association.

**<http://www.lupusresearch.org>**
Alliance for Lupus Research.

**<http://www.nih.gov/niams>**
National Institute of Arthritis and Musculoskeletal and Skin Diseases (NIAMS).

**<http://www.rheumatology.org>**
American College of Rheumatology.

# Glossary

**acupuncture**—An ancient form of treatment developed in Asia in which needles are placed in the body; used to help ease pain in people with arthritis.

**anemia**—A condition in which the number of red blood cells is below normal, making a person weak and tired.

**ankylosing spondylitis (AS)**—A form of inflammatory arthritis in which swelling occurs where the tendons and ligaments attach to the bone.

**antibodies**—Type of protein, made by the white blood cells, that protects the body by attacking invading germs.

**antigen**—A toxin or other substance to which the body reacts by producing antibodies.

**arthritis**—A disease that affects the joints.

**biofeedback**—A method of teaching patients how to relax their bodies by using a special machine.

**biologic agents**—Proteins that target chemicals in the body.

**bursa**—A small sac of fluid, near the joint, that lubricates the muscles.

**cartilage**—A thin layer of tough tissue that acts as a cushion on the end of each bone.

**corticosteroids**—Hormones, such as prednisone, that can quickly relieve pain and reduce swelling.

**COX-2 inhibitors**—A type of medication that reduces inflammation and eases pain; these drugs are thought to be easier on the stomach than some other pain-relievers.

**degenerative arthritis**—The most common type of arthritis, in which the cartilage is damaged.

**disease-modifying anti-rheumatic drugs (DMARDs)**—Drugs used to alter the course of a disease.

**double-blind test**—A test in which a real drug is given to one group of patients and a placebo is given to another group. Neither the people in the groups nor their doctors know who is taking which drug until the study ends.

**fibromyalgia**—A disease that affects the soft tissue around the joints and causes pain throughout the body.

**genes**—Tiny units within each cell that determine a person's traits.

**genetic marker**—A spot on a gene that only a certain number of people have. It can sometimes be used to predict who will get a certain disease.

**Heberden's nodes**—Bony knobs in the finger joints.

**HLA-B27**—A genetic marker linked to reactive arthritis and ankylosing spondylitis.

**HLA-DR4**—A genetic marker found in about 75 percent of those patients with rheumatoid arthritis.

**immune system**—The body's defense against germs and disease.

**inflammatory arthritis**—A type of arthritis marked by swelling and pain in the joints.

**juvenile rheumatoid arthritis (JRA)**—A form of inflammatory arthritis that strikes children.

**ligament**—Short bands of tough tissue that connect bones to other bones.

**lupus (systemic lupus erythematosus)**—An inflammatory disease that causes swollen joints and can affect muscles, skin, nerves, lungs, and other organs.

**Lyme disease**—An illness caused by tick bites that can lead to arthritis.

**macrophages**—Cells that eat invading germs.

**massage therapy**—An ancient form of treatment in which the muscles of the body are rubbed.

**methotrexate**—A DMARD used as a treatment for rheumatoid arthritis; also used for lupus and other inflammatory diseases and, in larger doses, for cancer.

**muscle**—Tissues that contract, moving the bones.

**nonsteroidal anti-inflammatory drugs (NSAIDs)**—Drugs that help reduce pain and swelling.

**osteoarthritis (OA)**—A form of degenerative arthritis in which the cartilage is damaged.

**pauciarticular JRA**—A type of juvenile rheumatoid arthritis that affects only one or two joints.

**pediatrician**—A doctor who specializes in caring for children.

**placebo**—A harmless substance used instead of a real medication.

**placebo effect**—A result in which a patient gets better because the patient believes the medication he or she is taking will help (even though the medication is a placebo).

**polyarticular JRA**—A type of juvenile rheumatoid arthritis that affects several joints.

**prednisone**—A type of steroid used to treat certain types of arthritis.

**reactive arthritis**—A type of arthritis thought to be caused by infection.

**remission**—A period of time when a person experiences no symptoms from a disease.

**rheumatoid arthritis (RA)**—A form of inflammatory arthritis that affects the synovial sac and can cause severe damage to the joints.

**rheumatoid factor**—A type of antibody found in the blood of about 80 percent of people with RA.

**rheumatologist**—A doctor who treats people with arthritis.

**sed rate**—A test that shows the speed at which red blood cells settle to the bottom of a tube. This test measures how active the arthritis is.

**seronegative spondyloarthropathy**—A type of disease that causes inflammation, especially in the spine and other joints. Reactive arthritis and ankylosing spondylitis are forms of seronegative spondyloarthropathy.

**suppressor cell**—A special type of white blood cell that signals the body to stop its attack on germs.

**synovial sac**—Thin tissue lining the joint and filled with fluid.

**systemic JRA**—A form of juvenile rheumatoid arthritis that affects the body's whole system. Still's disease is a form of systemic JRA.

**tendon**—Tough, fibrous bands of tissue that connect the muscles to the bones.

**TENS unit**—A device that emits a low-level electrical current, blocking pain signals to the brain.

**titanium**—A shiny, lightweight but strong metal that is used in joint replacements.

**tumor necrosis factor**—A chemical that causes inflammation in the joints.

**X-ray**—A band of electromagnetic waves that can be used to take pictures of internal structures of the body; a picture made by means of X-rays.

# Index